The Real (Hidden) Reasons Diets Have Failed You

15 Powerful Tools to Lose the Weight and Change Your Life - Diet FREE

Your fat is not your fault. Really! Diets fail. 97% of dieters regain all the weight in less than three years and blame themselves for it.
They shouldn't... and neither should you.

In this ground-breaking Itty Bitty® Book, Liz Bull shares her passion and expertise with you to gain valuable insight into the hidden reasons diets have failed you...and what you can do about them.

Liz gives you 15 concrete ways to take charge... identify the things which have been stopping your weight loss so that you can be naturally slim and NEVER diet again!

What her clients say:

- "I lost the weight without diet or willpower and my chronic migraines stopped."
- "Liz's holistic method delivers... more than I could have ever imagined...spiritual, physical and emotional. I am so grateful!"
- "My life is so different now. Some would call it a miracle...but I call it *The Liz Effect.*"

Isn't it time you went Diet FREE? Pick up a copy of this essential book today.

Your Amazing Itty Bitty® Diet FREE Weight Loss Book

15 Key Steps to a Body and a Life You Love

Elizabeth (Liz) Bull

Published by Itty Bitty® Publishing
A subsidiary of S & P Productions, Inc.

Printed in the United States of America

Itty Bitty® Publishing
311 Main Street, Suite D
El Segundo, CA 90245
(310) 640-8885

ISBN: 978-0-99875597-0-8

Dedication

This book is dedicated to the millions of women who have struggled with weight and body image, especially my Mom.

I am thankful to the many researchers, deep thinkers and practitioners who have dedicated themselves to unlocking the mysteries of weight gain, food-related illnesses and the profound psyche-soma relationship:

John Bradshaw
Dr. Robert Bull
Dr. Alan Christiansen
Dr. Peter D'Adamo
Dr. Beverly Goode-Kanawati
Dr. Sarah Gottfried
Louise Hay
Dr. Mark Hyman
Dr. Michael Lincoln
Dr. Bruce Lipton
Geneen Roth
Dr. Sanford Siegel
Caroline Sutherland
Doreen Virtue
Anthony William

Stop by our Itty Bitty® Publishing website to find interesting information regarding Diet Free Weight Loss.

www.IttyBittyPublishing.com

Or visit Liz at

www.lizbull.com

Follow Liz on Twitter
@lizbullVGB

Follow Liz on Facebook

Liz Bull

Table of Contents

Introduction

It's not your fault....really.

I get it. You have been struggling with weight for a long time. You have tried every diet and weight loss plan and nothing has worked for you.

This Itty Bitty® Book is for you if:

- You follow diets to the letter. Everyone else loses ten pounds. You lose one (maybe).
- You are sick of meetings. You turned your weight loss over to a higher power and nothing happened.
- You are sick of counting calories/carbohydrates/points.
- You are sick of weighing and measuring foods that you do not even like.
- You dread getting on a scale.
- You dread shopping for clothes.
- You are tired of feeling deprived and hungry.
- You hide in the back for group photos.
- You are tired of (expensive) food plan meals that taste like cardboard.
- Working out just wasn't working.
- Traditional "diet foods" leave you hungry.
- You suspect something is wrong with you.
- You find yourself hiding candy and cookie wrappers (and you live alone!).
- You find yourself staring into the fridge and have no idea what you really want.
- The idea of another weight loss program makes you want to scream or cry...or both.

And who wouldn't?

I get it. I grew up with a Mom who was morbidly obese...and I struggled with weight myself.
I just hated it when people would look at what I had on my plate. I felt so judged! Heck, I even judged myself.

My worst memory is the big family Thanksgiving dinner when Mom's brother offered her two chairs to sit on. I watched in horror as she choked back the tears. It really broke my heart.

My Mom tried everything... even a medically supervised fast. She would always regain the weight, a victim of the simple thinking that fewer calories in and more calories out would result in permanent weight loss. It never did.

This equation is a set up for failure and despair. I learned that it did not have to be this way. It is what this book is about. It is about the hidden reasons for weight and what you can do about them. My mission is to create a world where no woman goes to her grave still ashamed of and hating her body.

That includes you.

Step 1
Why Diets Don't Work

There are soooo many diets out there. You know.
You have tried many of them.... perhaps all of
them. And they did not work.

Why not? Why don't diets work for everybody?
Here's why.

1. We are all different... like snowflakes.
   Nutrition is not a "one-size-fits-all"
   situation, as anyone who has suffered
   from a food allergy will tell you.
2. Everyone's body has a different set-point
   for weight, designed to keep you safe.
3. Diets cause stress and higher cortisol
   levels. High cortisol levels cause leptin
   resistance, which in turn causes insulin
   resistance.
4. If your body wants to be fat (for its own
   reasons), dieting will only make it fatter.
5. If you are starving emotionally, your
   body will compensate for that with
   weight.
6. Your body is the boss. It has the last
   word on what it will do with the food.

TIP: Here Are Other Reasons Why Diets Fail:

- Emotional toxins cause stress and higher cortisol levels.
- Toxins, including medications, block the body's ability to burn fat.
- The things that force your body to lose weight are not the same things that get your body to want to be thin.
- Diets trick your body into thinking that there is a famine. Your body responds by retaining fat and makes more in order to keep you alive...the "starvation response."
- Sleep deprivation and sleep apnea cause chronic exhaustion and junk food cravings.
- Fat absorbs radiation. Your body will use the fat to protect you from it.
- Food additives, processed foods, artificial sweeteners and flavor enhancers like MSG cause hormonal chaos in your body.
- Nutritional starvation. If you are not eating foods that your body can digest and absorb, your body will hold on to fat.
- Epstein-Barr Virus effects.

Step 2
What's Reality Behind Weight:
Your Subconscious Mind

You may think that your conscious mind controls your life. It doesn't. It is your subconscious mind (your hidden beliefs/hurts/traumas) that control 90-95% of what you do. You must use kinesiology or muscle-testing to ferret these out. Learn how at www.lizbull.com.

Permanent weight loss results from:

1. Eliminating physical toxins
2. Eliminating emotional toxins
3. Revealing and shifting hidden beliefs which are causing your body to hold on to weight
4. Healing hidden hurts and traumas
5. Nourishing your body physically, emotionally and spiritually
6. Being well-hydrated
7. Establishing the eating habits of naturally thin people
8. Eating only when you are physically hungry; learning to identify your body's hunger signals
9. Identifying and countering your "head hunger"

TIP: Some common subconscious beliefs you may be experiencing:

- I need to be heavy to feel safe.
- Nothing works for me.
- If I'm thin, nobody will take me seriously.
- If I'm thin and sexy, I'll be raped or attacked… or feel unsafe around men.
- To be accepted by my family, I have to be fat…because they all are.
- If I'm thin, I'll be weak and I'll die.
- Being heavy will keep me from cheating.
- My weight helps me say, "no."
- If I lose this weight and pursue my dream and fail, then that will mean that there is something REALLY wrong with me. I won't be able to blame the weight.
- I won't know who I am if I'm thin.
- If I am thin and beautiful, people will think I'm superficial. Or that I must be a bitch.
- I have to eat everything so that Mommy will love me (or won't punish me).
- I have to eat FAST or I won't get enough.
- If I'm thin, Mom will be jealous.
- If I let myself eat fries, I won't ever stop.
- My body betrays me. I can't trust it.
- I need my fat to hide and be safe.

Step 3
Emotional Toxins – Hidden Hurts and Traumas

In my experience, every extra pound you carry on your body often equals a pound of emotional pain you're carrying in your heart.

1. Clearing the emotional pain allows for the release of the weight—easily and effortlessly.
2. In my experience with thousands of healings, overeating (as well as other physical ailments) is often triggered by emotionally painful traumas or situations.
3. Emotional pain and trauma often starts quite early in life... before the age of five...when you are still very vulnerable and impressionable....so you think that these things are your fault...or that you are just *wrong*.
4. To protect yourself, you bury these hurts in layers of fat.
5. To protect yourself, you bulk up to hide...or set boundaries.

TIP: Here are common characteristics:

- Perfectionistic: Often the first-born; trying to live up to high expectations.
- Mom frequently dieted; overemphasis on weight/appearance.
- Love was conditional or performance-based.
- Mom denied her own needs.
- Rigid discipline, severe punishment, physical and/or verbal abuse.
- Sexuality ignored or considered "dirty"; the body's existence and needs are wrong or inconvenient.
- Being used as parent's emotional support or confidante.
- Child forced to be adult—raising siblings, not allowed to be a child.
- Neglect: Child was ignored/unprotected.
- Parent addicted—alcohol, drugs, food!
- Family ignored or denied negative emotions; rage often present.
- Food/drink always used for pleasure or reward; emphasis on sweets and desserts.
- There was lots of criticism.
- Sexual abuse/fondling/inappropriate touching by family member/close friend.

Step 4
Fear

Fear is a key player keeping you fat.

Here are six of the most common fears:

1. The biggest is a fear of scarcity. Even fear of not having enough money can send a message to your body that,"We don't have enough... so save what we've got!" If you think, "I'd better eat now since I don't know when I'll get another chance"... it's fear.
2. Fear of being attacked. Fat can create a buffer.
3. Fear of the world. Fat becomes a convenient place to hide and retreat.
4. Fear of becoming too sexy and attracting unwanted attention from men (or women).
5. Fear of becoming weak and dying...or wasting away.
6. Fear of being hungry.

TIP: Here are some other fears which will keep weight in place:

- Fear of not being taken seriously. Often we associate "big" with being the boss and being respected.
- Fear of failure or making a mistake will often set up "head hunger"... especially for sweets... anything to soothe.
- Fear of being rejected by loved ones/friends because you have changed.
- Fear of losing sense of self and identity. Who will I be when I'm thin?
- Fear of becoming promiscuous, cheating on your mate. Often, weight has kept you safe from your desire to "fool around." Unfortunately, it often keeps you trapped in bad relationships.
- Fear of making the critics "right." You know, those people who have been telling you to lose weight. This is where your inner rebel comes out.
- Fear of jealousy from other women. How often have you heard the term "Skinny Bitch"?
- Fear of failure. You've been on a million diets and none of them worked. What if this doesn't work either? Forget it!

Step 5
Anger

Anger plays major role in weight... especially if it is something you have to *eat* or *stuff*.

Here are things you need to know about anger:

1. Anger raises blood pressure. When you say "He makes my blood boil"... it's true!
2. Anger raises the stress hormone cortisol.
3. You may have been taught that anger is bad, to not feel it or show it. You may use food to stuff it or express it instead.
4. Anger at yourself for past mistakes or poor decisions can add to weight. You may punish yourself with the weight.
5. Dieting may make you angry. You may hate the restriction, being told what to do, and having to be *good* all the time.
6. Anger at how unfair life is or how you have been treated can keep or add to weight. You may compensate with food.
7. Anger raises adrenalin levels.
8. Unresolved anger can lead to digestive problems, insomnia and headaches.
9. If you can't punch somebody or scream, you often eat!

TIP: Here are some things you can do to handle anger:

- Realize that anger is legitimate. When someone has crossed a boundary, you have the right to be angry about it.
- Acknowledge the feeling. Own it! You have the right to your feelings.
- Stop talking about what made you angry. Repeating it gives it energy.
- Move! Anger requires physical expression. It is an energy that moves through the body.
- Press your "pause" button! Take deep breaths until you calm down. Breathe in through your nose and out through your mouth.
- Punch the air or a pillow for 30 seconds.
- Stomp around; walk fast for 10 minutes.
- Walking daily calms anger and decreases blood pressure.
- Go someplace where you can scream.
- Tap on your collarbone or use EFT (Emotional Freedom Technique-Tapping).
- Write it down. Think of the person, the incident or the situation and use this formula to write: 1) all resentments; 2) all regrets; 3) all things not communicated. Then release it. Tear it up. Burn it. You get the idea.

Step 6
Tension

Tension has a huge effect on our ability to lose weight... as well as contributing to weight gain. Tension can also come from too many demands or demands you feel unable to meet.

1. Tension is when your system is "on alert" in anticipation of undefined threats.
2. Tension makes you crave carbohydrates.
3. Unresolved issues in relationships lead to tension and weight gain. Clean up or end relationships which are unsatisfying, draining, abusive or toxic.
4. Tension creates an overactive appetite.
5. Tension makes it harder to lose the fat.
6. Tension reduces digestion and impairs the immune system.
7. Poor digestion leads to the "starvation response."
8. Tension requires physical expression. Your muscles need to relax and stretch.

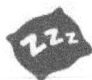

TIP: Here are tips to reduce tension:

- Stretch! Take a walk... anywhere will do. Stress needs movement.
- Getting enough Vitamin B12 can help with chronic tension.
- Drink Tension Tamer Tea during the day.
- Journal. Awareness is a critical part of weight loss. Use your journal to safely voice frustrations. My favorite format is to choose a subject/incident/person and write all 1) resentments; 2) regrets; 3) things not communicated. (Everything you would have loved to have said but couldn't/didn't.)
- Take a soak in the tub. Use lavender-scented bath salts.
- Get enough Magnesium. Being deficient actually causes chronic exhaustion and stress. I like Natural Vitality CALM, (magnesium supplement) taken at night.
- Meditate. There are excellent recorded meditations which take only 15 minutes. Slip on some headphones and relax.
- Breathe deeply and slowly 6 to 10 times.
- Dance! Skip! Hula hoop! Bounce!
- Color! Coloring books for grown-ups are great for reducing tension....and FUN!

Step 7
Shame

Everybody experiences some kind of shame; however, dieting promotes it! Shame is a combination of self-blame, self-doubt and low self-esteem. It is the intensely painful feeling or experience of believing that you are flawed (wrong) and therefore, unworthy and undeserving of love and belonging.

Shame is a huge factor in keeping you fat. For many of you, it started with the Clean Plate Club.

1. You are a member of this club if you have to: clean your plate at every meal; finish the bag of chips, bag of M&M's, cookies... you name it.
2. You are a member of the "Clean Plate Club," if you continue to hear: *"What about the starving children?"* or that killer, *"Waste not, want not!"*
3. In the Club, you have been conditioned into disconnecting and ignoring your body's signals that you are full.
4. Club members are anxious about leaving food on the plate or throwing food away.

TIP: Shame occurs because we are constantly bombarded with uber-perfect models for just about everything.

Here are some other thoughts you may have that are indicators of shame:

- I had a soda today. I'm such a failure.
- I never stick to anything. I'm such a loser.
- I have no self-control.
- There's nothing to like about my body.
- I'm so ashamed that I cheated on my finals, mate, etc. I deserve to be fat.
- No one will love me until I'm thin.
- I feel icky (and a bit violated) when someone compliments me.
- Feeling sexy is shameful and wrong.
- I have to be heavy to be a good girl.
- If I look after my own needs and my body, someone else will suffer.
- What I want doesn't matter.
- I don't matter.
- I don't have what it takes to succeed.
- I hate myself.
- I hate my thighs/breasts/eyes/hair, etc.
- I can never get anything right.
- I'm just ugly.
- It's my fault that I'm so fat.

Step 8
Food Sensitivities
When Healthy Food Isn't Healthy

When your body has a food sensitivity, that food is toxic to you. It cannot process that particular food and usually has an adverse reaction to it. Food sensitivities can provoke hunger.

1. Common reactions are stuffy nose, bloating, rashes, post-nasal drip, sneezing, achy joints, water retention, hunger and sleepiness.
2. Sometimes the reaction is more severe, like chronic indigestion and heartburn or even life-threatening anaphylactic shock.
3. Many of you are used to tolerating discomfort in your bodies, not realizing that it is related to food. Many so-called, "healthy" foods may be holding your body hostage, promoting insulin resistance and causing weight gain.
4. When your body cannot digest and use a particular food, this sets up a starvation response and provokes a vicious cycle.
5. Many sensitivities are related to blood type. Read Dr. Peter D'Adamo's **Eat Right 4 Your Type.**

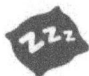

TIP: To find out which foods are best for *your* body, learn how to muscle test (kinesiology)at www.lizbull.com.

This uses your body's inner wisdom. Or get an ALCAT test.

The following foods are always problematic:

- Sugar. Causes unstable blood sugar.
- High Fructose Corn Syrup
- MSG (Monosodium Glutamate) and free glutamates, in 80% of processed foods.
- Artificial Sweeteners. Aspartame is toxic to the brain, addictive, desensitizes the tongue sweetness, causes weight gain. Sucralose is chlorine added to glucose.

These foods can, surprisingly, be problematic:

- Soy. It affects hormones and thyroid.
- Dairy. It sets off inflammation.
- Eggs. May be the yolk or the white.
- Corn. Pro-inflammatory.
- Peanuts...and other legumes/beans.
- Wheat and grains (not just gluten).
- Many fruits - citrus in particular.
- Nightshade family vegetables.
- Many spices, herbs, condiments and fermented foods.
- Many nuts.

Step 9
Physical Toxins

Physical Toxins profoundly affect weight and your efforts to lose weight. Here are things you need to know:

1. Toxins are potentially harmful elements, molecules or organisms that your body must either eliminate or store in a "safe" place. Toxins come from our environment: food, water, air, electricity, radiation, water supply, medication*, food additives, preservatives and artificial sweeteners. Toxins can block your body's capacity to burn fat, cause inflammation and exacerbate insulin resistance. (*All medications are toxic to the body in some way. Only take drugs when absolutely necessary. Find natural alternatives whenever possible.)
2. Fat protects you from toxins. It encapsulates them. It takes the load off of the liver, whose job it is to be the sewage plant for your body.
3. Heavy Metals. Many people are carrying heavy metals. Get tested.
4. Yeast or candida feeds on sugar and robs your body of nutrients.

TIP: Here are ways to eliminate physical toxins:

- Heavy metals can be cleaned out with greens: chlorella, parsley or cilantro. Seaweeds and chia seeds will also bind up the fat soluble toxins for clearing out. Vitamin C (½ lemon in some hot water) also helps.
- If you have a pet, you probably have parasites. There are several excellent parasite cleanses on the market. They do need to be used in a particular sequence, allowing time for the initial die-off and then the emergence of the eggs. The second round then kills off the newly born critters.
- Yeast cleanses are available at Whole Foods and health food stores or online. The essential ingredient is the herb (actually from a tree) Pau D'Arco.
- Eating more live, fresh, organic foods will reduce the inflow of toxins to the body. The extra fiber will clear out the colon of stagnant waste and undigested food. The enzymes will aid digestion.
- Drinking enough water daily to flush out the toxins.

Step 10
Gut Health, Digestion, Enzymes and Bacteria

Gut health and proper digestion are crucial for maintaining your body's ideal weight. When your body is not assimilating nutrients, it is literally starving.

1. Many of you suffer from poor digestion and ammonia permeability.
2. Modern farming has depleted many of the nutrients, friendly bacteria and plant-based microbes essential for proper digestion and assimilation of nutrients that used to be in food. Modern food processing destroys even more of the much-needed nutrients.
3. Digestive enzymes break down foods into their nutritional components so that the body can assimilate them. If you are deficient in these enzymes, you can't extract the nutrients. This means that you have to eat more in order to get enough to truly nourish your body.
4. Cooking changes the chemistry of food.
5. Digestion actually starts in your mouth.
6. Poor dental health inhibits good digestion and absorption of nutrients.

TIP: Here are some ways to improve gut health:

- Chewing each bite slowly and mindfully 30 times will start the digestive process properly.
- Grains and dairy are digested best when you eat them AFTER the meat. This also slows down the rate at which the sugar in them is released into your bloodstream.
- If you have ever taken antibiotics, you need to take a course of probiotics to replenish your intestinal tract with friendly bacteria.
- Avoid processed foods. They are nutritionally deficient. The preservatives in them kill enzymes.
- Your stomach acid necessary to digest properly may be depleted. Rebuild it by drinking 16 ounces of fresh celery juice each morning on an empty stomach.
- Eat proteins earlier in the day/mid-day, when your digestive system is at its peak.
- Eat carbohydrates later in the day/evening, when the system is entering "rest" mode.
- Filter chlorinated water. Chlorine destroys the microorganisms and friendly bacteria in your digestive system.

Step 11
Water

Starvation is not just about food. It is also about water.

1. Your body is about 70% water.
2. Water is essential to life. You can go longer without food than without water.
3. Sodas, tea and coffee will never provide what your body actually needs.
4. Chlorinated tap water kills the friendly bacteria in your digestive system.
5. Having enough water is essential to the digestive process and for eliminating waste. If you are having problems with constipation, it is likely that you are not getting enough water.
6. Thirst often masquerades as a craving for sweets/soft drinks.
7. When you don't drink enough water, your body can't cool itself when necessary.
8. Drinking room temperature water between meals helps flush out food particles.
9. Water is needed to carry nutrients from the stomach into the intestine walls, improving absorption.
10. Water helps the body remove toxins, both through the skin and the kidneys.

TIP: Here are things you need to know to get enough good water:

- Start the day with a glass of warm water. I like to add a 1/2 fresh lemon/lime to this. It helps to detoxify your body.
- Drink two glasses of water before each meal.
- The ideal amount of water to consume daily is one ounce for every 2.2 pounds (1 Kilo) of body weight.
- Drink water to curb nighttime hunger.
- Use filtered water if your water supply is chlorinated.
- If you are craving sweets or soft drinks, grab a glass of water.
- Keep water handy on your desk, in your car/truck...wherever you work.
- Drink water instead of coffee or tea on your commute to work or school.
- Drink sparkling water instead of alcoholic beverages at parties. Many of them have added minerals which are good for your body. Alcohol dehydrates your body.
- Avoid "sports drinks."
- Avoid drinking water from plastic bottles.

Step 12
Hormones

Hormones play a huge role in regulating weight.

1. Hormones are your body's chemical messengers, and they control just about every physiological process in your body. They regulate metabolism, activate your immune system, affect your reproduction cycle, etc.
2. Some women go through menopause with no side effects or discomfort. For most, it is an emotional and physical transition. HRT (Hormone Replacement Therapy) can adversely affect weight loss.
3. When your hormones are out of whack, you can feel depressed and lethargic and, as a result, become prone to self-medicating with food. This becomes a vicious cycle, as the foods themselves can throw your hormones off balance, causing you to crave more foods that will further throw off your hormonal balance.

TIP: Here are some additional things you should know.

- Avoid coffee, a go-to food when you are feeling lethargic or sluggish. It can wreak havoc on your endocrine system, which will cause you to feel even more sluggish.
- NASA identified caffeine as the chemical most responsible for human error. Avoid it.
- The thyroid gland controls the rate at which you use energy. Thyroid problems impair weight loss. An estimated 10 million women have an undiagnosed thyroid problem caused by Epstein Baarr virus. Get Sanford Siegel's book, **Is Your Thyroid Making You Fat?** Or familiarize yourself with Dr. Alan Christianson's and Anthony William's work **Medical Medium**.
- Your adrenal glands produce excess cortisol in response to tension.
- Tension creates an overactive appetite for carbohydrates.
- When cortisol rises, blood sugar levels go crazy. Digestion is impaired.
- Insulin resistance can keep serotonin from reaching your brain, causing sleep problems.
- Constant stress causes adrenal fatigue.
- Read Dr. Sara Gottfried's book **The Hormone Cure** for more information.

Step 13
Stress

Stress is a key reason you are unable to lose weight. It raises cortisol levels. Here are some of the top reasons for stress:

1. As a woman, you are really prone to this. Your natural urge to nurture and please is your undoing. The result is that you take on others' "stuff" at your expense.
2. You are bombarded by impossible expectations. Instead of choosing what would actually serve you best, you say, "Oh sure, I'll do that!"
3. Much of what you do does not actually need to be done. Baking cupcakes for the entire class IS optional! So is folding your teenager's laundry.
4. A need to control creates stress. Much of what you do could be done by someone else. They may not do it the same way you would do it, but it would get done. If you find yourself rearranging the dishes in the dishwasher, stop it.
5. Over-scheduling the day.
6. Failure or forgetting to schedule time to rest and renew. You both need and deserve it!

TIP: Here are ways to stop stress:

- Just say, "NO." Clear your plate of all the activities that don't really serve you. Only YOU get to decide what those are.
- To every request, ask if this, "one more thing" would enhance your life or add to your stress. If just asking this question makes your jaw tighten or your shoulders hunch a bit, then the answer is, "NO."
- Practice the art of the gentle decline! Say this: "**Gee**, you know, my plate is totally full right now **and** I'm really flattered that you thought of me. I wish you luck in finding the right person to do this." Be sure to say "AND" not "BUT." IMPORTANT! Do NOT apologize!! Say "GEE" or "GOSH", not "Sorry."
- Look at what you are now doing that adds to your stress… and STOP it.
- Choose the three most important things to do each day. Concentrate on those.
- Give yourself some gold stars and take a little break when they are done.
- Carve out "me-time" and put it on your calendar... sacred time to do whatever feeds your spirit and soul.
- Have a nice cup of tea, preferably with a friend. Try Tension Tamer Tea.
- Breathe. Breathe in through your nose and out through your mouth...about five times to instantly calm down. Ah-h-h.

Step 14
Real (Physical) Hunger vs. Head Hunger
vs. Thirst

Hunger is... complicated! Everybody experiences what they think is hunger. The problem is that often, they are being tricked or confused! The mere look of certain foods may make you salivate. Advertizers use this. You may associate certain foods with comfort. This is "head hunger." You are taught to be "hungry" at certain times of the day... fitting into someone else's schedule rather than honoring your own body's signals.

You have been trained to confuse "clean plate" with *full* when *full* happened long before the plate was clean... and plates are 51% larger than in the 1900's. Here are the facts about hunger:

1. Food can never satisfy hunger which is not physical.
2. Physical hunger comes with signals. First, a little gnawing in your stomach. Then, slight hunger pangs and eventually some growling.
3. Diet FREE means eating when you are physically hungry and stopping at *full*.

TIP: Knowing the difference between head hunger, physical hunger and thirst:

- Head Hunger happens instantly; it wants carbohydrates and soothing.
- Head Hunger often persists as an empty feeling in the stomach, even after eating.
- Head Hunger may actually be fatigue. So, take a break or have a nap.
- Head Hunger may be a need for fresh air. Get some.
- Head Hunger may be a need for a hug or some self-care. Give yourself the space to figure out *what* is going on. Ask, what is it that I *really* want?
- Often you mistake hunger for thirst. So, grab a glass of water first.
- You are often not nearly as hungry as you think. The first three bites of food, chewed thoroughly, are the most satisfying. Stop and ask, "Am I still hungry?" before eating more.
- You may be susceptible to suggestion and social pressure...over-riding your body's *full* signal. If you ordered dessert because your friend did or finished a dish in order to spare someone's feelings, learn to say: "I just can't eat another bite." or "May I take this home for later?" or "No, thanks."

Step 15
Sleep

Sleep is essential for well-being. If you have interrupted sleep, you become chronically exhausted. This puts stress on your body. Here are some things you should know:

1. 90% of your fat-burning happens when the body is at rest, not in the gym.
2. Often you eat because you are tired.
3. Chronic fatigue may be due to sleep apnea. Get checked.
4. Chronic fatigue causes junk food cravings.
5. Chronic Fatigue Syndrome is linked to Epstein-Barr virus. Read more about this in **Medical Medium**.
6. Remember that your body needs 8 to 10 hours of sleep to function properly.
7. Fat-burning happens at the end of the sleep cycle.

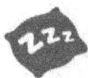

TIP: Here are some suggestions to get better sleep.

- Cut down on hard to digest foods (like meat) at night. Eat most of your daily carbohydrates (more easily digested) in the evening.
- Stop eating 3 hours before bedtime.
- Unplug! Keep electronics out of the bedroom. Their lights disrupt sleep.
- Avoid caffeine and alcohol.
- Have a routine. Lay out your clothes, car keys, briefcase, etc. Pack your lunch.
- Take a nice hot, relaxing bath with lavender-scented bath salts.
- To clear your head, write down your worries and plan your day.
- Make the bedroom cool, dark and quiet.
- Optimal temperature for sleep is between 62F and 72F degrees.
- Use black-out shades if needed.
- Consider a nightcap of Natural Vitality CALM. The magnesium relaxes muscles.
- Consider a nightcap of Chamomile Tea.
- Go to bed before 11PM. Your body's hard-wired repair schedule starts around 10PM.
- Spritz some lavender on your pillow.
- Meditate.
- Get enough Vitamin D.

You've finished. Before you go...

Tweet/share that you finished this book.

Please star rate this book.

Reviews are solid gold to writers. Please take a few minutes to give us some itty bitty feedback.

ABOUT THE AUTHOR

Liz Bull helps women who are fed up with weight loss programs that don't work to finally get a body and a life they love. A veteran and "survivor" of restrictive diets, she cracked the code and is now dedicated to helping women everywhere discover the hidden reasons for their weight, heal emotional eating, reach their healthy weight, and to look and feel fabulous and feminine. In this book, she busts up the myths, misconceptions and misinformation about obesity...disconnecting *fault* from *fat*.

Her holistic signature private coaching program (Diet-FREE Weight Loss™) and articles teach women a natural, sustainable and joyous approach to weight loss. She works with clients to identify and clear the root causes for the weight... so they end the battle with their body, lose weight and never diet again.

A Certified Virtual Gastric Band Practitioner, Liz has long been fascinated by the important role hidden beliefs play in our lives, especially with weight. She is also a Medical Intuitive and Master Theta Healer. Her other studies and certifications include EFT (Tapping), Psych-K, Matrix Energetics, Access Consciousness, Qi Gong, NLP, Biofield Healing, Full Spectrum Healing and Transcendental Meditation.

She is a regular contributor to Eydis magazine and a member of the Obesity Action Coalition.

**If you enjoyed this Itty Bitty® book
You might also enjoy…**

- **Your Amazing Itty Bitty® Weight Loss Book** – Suzy Prudden and Joan Meijer-Hirschland

- **Your Amazing Itty Bitty® Self-Esteem Book** – Jade Elizabeth

- **Your Amazing Itty Bitty® Heal Your Body Book** – Patricia Garza Pinto

  Or any of our other Itty Bitty® Books available online.

www.ingramcontent.com/pod-product-compliance
Lightning Source LLC
Chambersburg PA
CBHW071344290326
41933CB00040B/2237